THIS BOOK BELONGS TO:

....

....

....

....

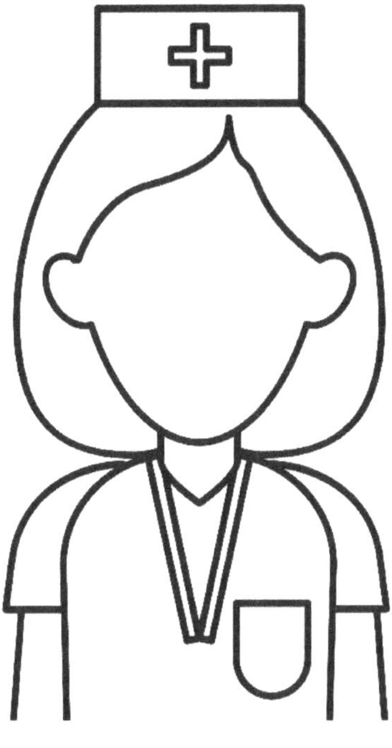

www.ingramcontent.com/pod-product-compliance
Lightning Source LLC
Chambersburg PA
CBHW070416220526
45466CB00004B/1428
* 9 7 8 1 6 9 6 8 7 4 7 1 7 *